Consider *The Sacred Woman Journal* as an opportunity to explore the pathways of time and record your experiences each day, chronicling your own road map to self-enlightenment and revealing the indwelling Mystery of the Hidden Sun.

On each page, you will find an invitation to awaken the healer within. Recite the Sacred Word Meditation atop each sheet. The lines that follow are your Sacred Space for recording your thoughts, experiences, visions, and desires, bringing life to your soul and clarity to your mind.

Spend time daily journaling, making note of the hourly guides for channeling inner vision (before dawn), activation (midday), inner reflection (sunset), and rest (evening). As you travel through each Gateway, ascending to your brightest inner light, these rituals will help take away your broken heart and your wounded life. Expect that as you travel through each Gateway, freedom, unbreakable peace, overflowing joy, love, forgiveness, and new beginnings will be at your beck and call.

At the opening of each week, you will find space to track your daily practices, from inversion and hydrotherapy to meals and water intake. As you mindfully observe your work and harmonize with the various systems of wellness, you will affirm your sense of well-being and ascend to your brightest inner light. These checklists serve as a guide, an invitation to complete the practices that resonate and will help you along your journey to healing and revitalization. You might not complete every item every day, and that is okay. And if you need, you can always return to the pages of *Sacred Woman* for additional insights into each activity.

Like the flow of a river, your questions will pour into answers. Tap into your inner scribe and blossom into beauty, grace, and wellness. Every day and on every page, through every word written, your mind, body, and spirit will direct you along a path of liberation.

The Most High, the Ancient Ones, the Shining Beings, the Ancestors, and the Elders walk with you daily, giving you knowledge of self with each stroke of your pen.

PREPARATION FOR
SACRED WOMAN JOURNALING

Trust and know that all that you need is inside of you. Peacefully go within; light your candle, burn your incense, drink your herbal tea from a bowl of complete wholeness. Breathe deeply, live your prayers, then channel your new life. In the spirit of the seer, the knower, the watcher, channel your Inner Vision Treasure Chest, which is the Gateway to peace on Earth and goodwill to humanity.

Mer (love), and *Ra* (light),
Queen Afua

THE SACRED WOMAN JOURNAL

QUEEN AFUA ✦ *The Velvet Sword*

✦ EIGHTY-FOUR DAYS ✦
OF REFLECTION AND HEALING

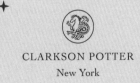

CLARKSON POTTER
New York

Published in the United States by Clarkson Potter, an imprint of Random House, a division of Penguin Random House LLC, New York.

CLARKSON POTTER and colophon are registered trademarks of Penguin Random House LLC.

Based on *Sacred Woman Healing Journal* (One World/Random House, 2016).

Editor: Porscha Burke
Designer: Lise Sukhu
Production Editor: Serena Wang
Production Manager: Luisa Francavilla
Compositor: Margaret Discenza, Dix, Zoe Tokushige
Marketer: Brianne Sperber
Publicist: Lindsey Kennedy
Copy Editor: Nancy Tan

ISBN 978-0-593-23597-3

Printed in China

clarksonpotter.com
randomhousebooks.com

1 2 3 4 5 6 7 8 9

For the Global Sacred Woman Village Rites of Passage or Practitioner Program, books, and DVDs, contact (888) 344-4325 or visit www.QueenAfua.com or www.facebook.com/queenafua.

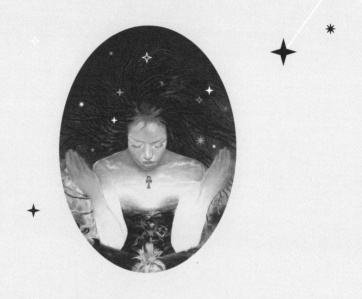

THIS JOURNAL BELONGS TO:

_____

_____

SACRED WOMAN PRAYER

Sacred Spirit, hold me near, close to your bosom.

Protect me from all harm and fear, beneath the stones of life.

Direct my steps in the right way as I journey through this vision.

Sacred Spirit, surround me in your absolutely perfect light.

Anoint me in your sacred purity; give me peace and divine insight.

Bless me, truly bless me, as I share this sacred life.

Teach me, Sacred Spirit, to be in tune with the Universe.

Teach me how to heal with the inner and outer elements

of air, fire, water, and earth.

CONTENTS

YOUR SACRED
WOMAN HEALING JOURNAL

It's like your mother . . .
loving and supportive.

It's like your wise teacher . . .
broadening your cipher in life.

It's like your closest and best girlfriend . . .
always there for you.

It's like your spiritual guide . . .
compassionate and nonjudgmental.

It's like your confidant . . .
honoring your secrets.

May your Sacred Woman healing journal
aid you in honoring the many parts of yourself that make you whole.

THE HEALER'S CREED
FROM THE MOTHERS OF ANTIQUITY
(Papyrus of Ani)

I am the woman who lightens the darkness.

I have come to lighten the darkness;

It is lightened.

I have overcome the destroyers.

I am there for those who weep, who hide their faces, who are sunk down.

They looked upon me then.

I am a Woman.

I am a Healer.

NUT CONSCIOUSNESS

DAYS 1–7

Sacred Womb Hour of Power Daily Checklist

DAY	1	2	3	4	5	6	7
4 – 6 a.m. *Nebt-Het Hour of Power* — **Journal Time for Channeling Your Inner Vision**							
Inversion (Elevate Legs on 3 Pillows)							
Hydrotherapy (Shower/Bath, Brush Teeth, Enema)							
Spiritual Observances 1–14 in the *Sacred Woman* Text for This Gateway							
Womb Yoga Fitness							
Liquid Breakfast (Freshly Pressed Fruit Juice)							
Solid Breakfast							
Herbal Tonic (Womb Care Love Herbal Detox Formula)							
Drink Water Intake: 16 oz.							

12 – 2 p.m. *Ast Hour of Power* — Journal Time for Activation

Liquid Lunch (Freshly Pressed Green Juice)							
Solid Vegan Lunch							
Meditation							
Drink Water Intake: 16 oz.							

You might not complete every item every day.
These checklists serve as a guide, an invitation to complete
the practices that resonate and will help you along
your journey to healing and revitalization.

DAY	1	2	3	4	5	6	7
4 – 6 p.m. *Het-Heru Hour of Power* — Journal Time for Inner Reflection							
Liquid Dinner							
Solid Vegan Dinner							
Home Detox							
Drink Water Intake: 16 oz.							
8 – 10 p.m. *Nut Hour of Power* — Journal Time for Rest							
Healing Bath +							
Clay Application ++							
Drink Water Intake: 16 oz.							
Inversion (Elevate Legs on 3 Pillows)							
Bed Rest							

+ FOR 30 MINUTES, SOAK IN BATH WITH EPSOM OR DEAD SEA SALT.

++ APPLY WITH GAUZE; KEEP ON OVERNIGHT.

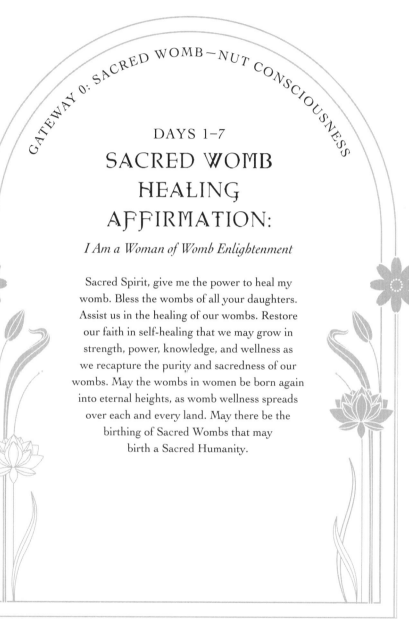

DAYS 1–7

SACRED WOMB HEALING AFFIRMATION:

I Am a Woman of Womb Enlightenment

Sacred Spirit, give me the power to heal my womb. Bless the wombs of all your daughters. Assist us in the healing of our wombs. Restore our faith in self-healing that we may grow in strength, power, knowledge, and wellness as we recapture the purity and sacredness of our wombs. May the wombs in women be born again into eternal heights, as womb wellness spreads over each and every land. May there be the birthing of Sacred Wombs that may birth a Sacred Humanity.

Gateway 0: Sacred Womb

"I am that I am on my journey to womb wellness.
My womb is sacred and so is my life."

DAY 1
Sacred Womb Wellness Day

4 – 6 a.m. Nebt-Het Hour — Journal Time for Channeling Your Inner Vision

_____

_____

12 – 2 p.m. Ast Hour — Journal Time for Activation

_____

_____

4 – 6 p.m. Het-Heru Hour — Journal Time for Inner Reflection

_____

_____

8 – 10 p.m. Nut Hour — Journal Time for Rest

_____

_____

Gateway 0: Sacred Womb

"I am that I am on my journey to womb wellness.
My womb is sacred and so is my life."

DAY 2
Sacred Womb Wellness Day

4 – 6 a.m. Nebt-Het Hour — Journal Time for Channeling Your Inner Vision

_____

_____

12 – 2 p.m. Ast Hour — Journal Time for Activation

_____

_____

4 – 6 p.m. Het-Heru Hour — Journal Time for Inner Reflection

_____

_____

8 – 10 p.m. Nut Hour — Journal Time for Rest

_____

_____

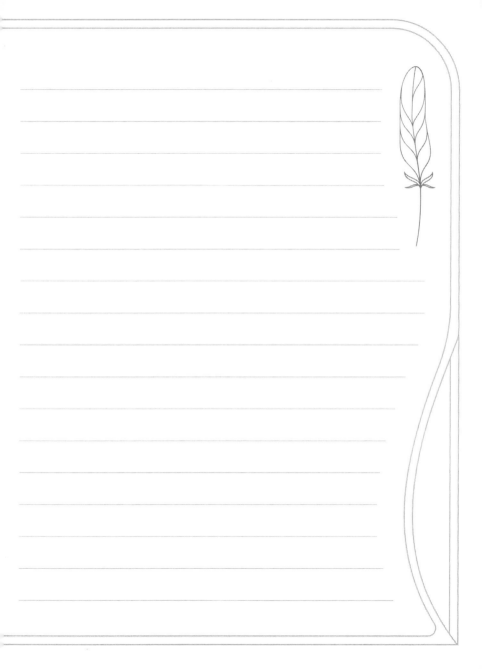

Gateway 0: Sacred Womb

"I am that I am on my journey to womb wellness.
My womb is sacred and so is my life."

DAY 3
Sacred Womb Wellness Day

4 – 6 a.m. Nebt-Het Hour — Journal Time for Channeling Your Inner Vision

_____

_____

12 – 2 p.m. Ast Hour — Journal Time for Activation

_____

_____

4 – 6 p.m. Het-Heru Hour — Journal Time for Inner Reflection

_____

_____

8 – 10 p.m. Nut Hour — Journal Time for Rest

_____

_____

Gateway 0: Sacred Womb

"I am that I am on my journey to womb wellness.
My womb is sacred and so is my life."

DAY 4
Sacred Womb Wellness Day

4 – 6 a.m. Nebt-Het Hour — Journal Time for Channeling Your Inner Vision

12 – 2 p.m. Ast Hour — Journal Time for Activation

4 – 6 p.m. Het-Heru Hour — Journal Time for Inner Reflection

8 – 10 p.m. Nut Hour — Journal Time for Rest

Gateway 0: Sacred Womb

"I am that I am on my journey to womb wellness.
My womb is sacred and so is my life."

DAY 5
Sacred Womb Wellness Day

4 – 6 a.m. Nebt-Het Hour — Journal Time for Channeling Your Inner Vision

_____

_____

12 – 2 p.m. Ast Hour — Journal Time for Activation

_____

_____

4 – 6 p.m. Het-Heru Hour — Journal Time for Inner Reflection

_____

_____

8 – 10 p.m. Nut Hour — Journal Time for Rest

_____

_____

Gateway 0: Sacred Womb

"I am that I am on my journey to womb wellness.
My womb is sacred and so is my life."

DAY 6
Sacred Womb Wellness Day

4 – 6 a.m. Nebt-Het Hour — Journal Time for Channeling Your Inner Vision

_____

_____

12 – 2 p.m. Ast Hour — Journal Time for Activation

_____

_____

4 – 6 p.m. Het-Heru Hour — Journal Time for Inner Reflection

_____

_____

8 – 10 p.m. Nut Hour — Journal Time for Rest

_____

_____

Gateway 0: Sacred Womb

"I am that I am on my journey to womb wellness.
My womb is sacred and so is my life."

DAY 7
Sacred Womb Wellness Day

4 – 6 a.m. Nebt-Het Hour—Journal Time for Channeling Your Inner Vision

_____

_____

12 – 2 p.m. Ast Hour—Journal Time for Activation

_____

_____

4 – 6 p.m. Het-Heru Hour—Journal Time for Inner Reflection

_____

_____

8 – 10 p.m. Nut Hour—Journal Time for Rest

_____

_____

TEHUTI CONSCIOUSNESS

DAYS 8–14

Sacred Word Hour of Power Daily Checklist

DAY	8	9	10	11	12	13	14
4 – 6 a.m. *Nebt-Het Hour of Power* — Journal Time for Channeling Your Inner Vision							
Inversion (Elevate Legs on 3 Pillows)							
Hydrotherapy (Shower/Bath, Brush Teeth, Enema)							
Spiritual Observances 1–14 in the *Sacred Woman* Text for This Gateway							
Womb Yoga Fitness							
Liquid Breakfast (Freshly Pressed Fruit Juice)							
Solid Breakfast							
Herbal Tonic (Womb Care Love Herbal Detox Formula)							
Drink Water Intake: 16 oz.							

12 – 2 p.m. *Ast Hour of Power* — Journal Time for Activation

Liquid Lunch (Freshly Pressed Green Juice)							
Solid Vegan Lunch							
Meditation							
Drink Water Intake: 16 oz.							

You might not complete every item every day.
These checklists serve as a guide, an invitation to complete the
practices that resonate and will help you along
your journey to healing and revitalization.

DAY	8	9	10	11	12	13	14

4 – 6 p.m. *Het-Heru Hour of Power* — Journal Time for Inner Reflection

	8	9	10	11	12	13	14
Liquid Dinner							
Solid Vegan Dinner							
Home Detox							
Drink Water Intake: 16 oz.							

8 – 10 p.m. *Nut Hour of Power* — Journal Time for Rest

	8	9	10	11	12	13	14
Healing Bath [+]							
Clay Application [++]							
Drink Water Intake: 16 oz.							
Inversion (Elevate Legs on 3 Pillows)							
Bed Rest							

[+] FOR 30 MINUTES, SOAK IN BATH WITH EPSOM OR DEAD SEA SALT.

[++] APPLY WITH GAUZE; KEEP ON OVERNIGHT.

DAYS 8–14

SACRED WORD HEALING AFFIRMATION:

I Am a Woman of Divine Intelligence

Sacred Spirit, assist me in speaking words of power.
May my words be anointed. May my words not
damage a soul. Sacred Spirit, help me to speak
words that heal, words that empower, words that
build, and words that transform. Help me to guard
my words so no venom passes my lips and no
destruction results from my speech. Rather, may
my words impart light to souls who are seeking
your face. If my words show me to be out of divine
right order, may my mind and mouth be cleansed.
Help me not to speak words that break down the
Divine in me or in my sister or my brother, my
mate, my child, my elders, or my ancestors. Sacred
Spirit, place words upon my lips that make my voice
disperse lotus blossoms. May my words be Sacred
Medicine that encourages all the souls I meet to
reach for greater heights. May my words speak
with your breath and sing your sweet song of life.
Because of the words and the evolved tones that I
utter, may goodness follow me all the days of my life.

Gateway 1: Sacred Word

"On my journey to the word of wisdom."

DAY 8
Sacred Word Medicine Day

4 – 6 a.m. Nebt-Het Hour—Journal Time for Channeling Your Inner Vision

12 – 2 p.m. Ast Hour—Journal Time for Activation

4 – 6 p.m. Het-Heru Hour—Journal Time for Inner Reflection

8 – 10 p.m. Nut Hour—Journal Time for Rest

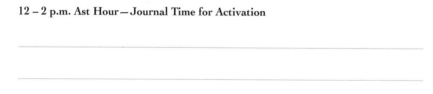

Gateway 1: Sacred Word

"On my journey to the word of wisdom."

DAY 9
Sacred Word Medicine Day

4 – 6 a.m. Nebt-Het Hour — Journal Time for Channeling Your Inner Vision

---

---

12 – 2 p.m. Ast Hour — Journal Time for Activation

---

4 – 6 p.m. Het-Heru Hour — Journal Time for Inner Reflection

---

8 – 10 p.m. Nut Hour — Journal Time for Rest

Gateway 1: Sacred Word

"On my journey to the word of wisdom."

DAY 10
Sacred Word Medicine Day

4 – 6 a.m. Nebt-Het Hour — Journal Time for Channeling Your Inner Vision

12 – 2 p.m. Ast Hour — Journal Time for Activation

4 – 6 p.m. Het-Heru Hour — Journal Time for Inner Reflection

8 – 10 p.m. Nut Hour — Journal Time for Rest

Gateway 1: Sacred Word

"On my journey to the word of wisdom."

DAY 11
Sacred Word Medicine Day

4 – 6 a.m. Nebt-Het Hour — Journal Time for Channeling Your Inner Vision

12 – 2 p.m. Ast Hour — Journal Time for Activation

4 – 6 p.m. Het-Heru Hour — Journal Time for Inner Reflection

8 – 10 p.m. Nut Hour — Journal Time for Rest

Gateway 1: Sacred Word

"On my journey to the word of wisdom."

DAY 12
Sacred Word Medicine Day

4 – 6 a.m. Nebt-Het Hour — Journal Time for Channeling Your Inner Vision

12 – 2 p.m. Ast Hour — Journal Time for Activation

4 – 6 p.m. Het-Heru Hour — Journal Time for Inner Reflection

8 – 10 p.m. Nut Hour — Journal Time for Rest

Gateway 1: Sacred Word

"On my journey to the word of wisdom."

DAY 13
Sacred Word Medicine Day

4 – 6 a.m. Nebt-Het Hour — Journal Time for Channeling Your Inner Vision

12 – 2 p.m. Ast Hour — Journal Time for Activation

4 – 6 p.m. Het-Heru Hour — Journal Time for Inner Reflection

8 – 10 p.m. Nut Hour — Journal Time for Rest

Gateway 1: Sacred Word

"On my journey to the word of wisdom."

DAY 14
Sacred Word Medicine Day

4 – 6 a.m. Nebt-Het Hour — Journal Time for Channeling Your Inner Vision

12 – 2 p.m. Ast Hour — Journal Time for Activation

4 – 6 p.m. Het-Heru Hour — Journal Time for Inner Reflection

8 – 10 p.m. Nut Hour — Journal Time for Rest

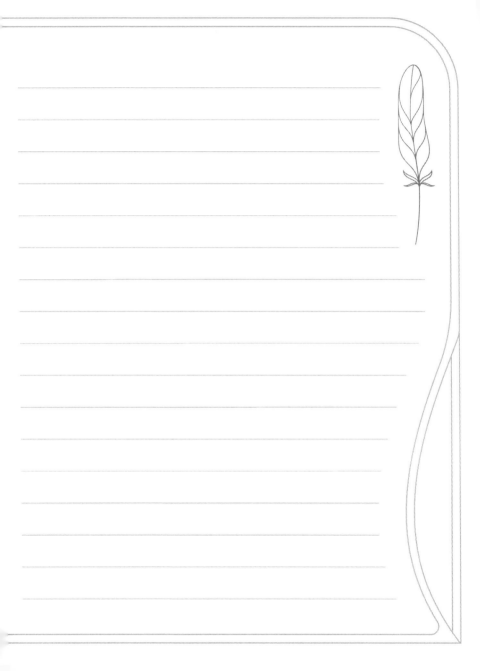

TA-URT CONSCIOUSNESS

DAYS 15–21

Sacred Food Hour of Power Daily Checklist

DAY	15	16	17	18	19	20	21

4 – 6 a.m. *Nebt-Het Hour of Power* — **Journal Time for Channeling Your Inner Vision**

	15	16	17	18	19	20	21
Inversion (Elevate Legs on 3 Pillows)							
Hydrotherapy (Shower/Bath, Brush Teeth, Enema)							
Spiritual Observances 1–14 in the *Sacred Woman* Text for This Gateway							
Womb Yoga Fitness							
Liquid Breakfast (Freshly Pressed Fruit Juice)							
Solid Breakfast							
Herbal Tonic (Womb Care Love Herbal Detox Formula)							
Drink Water Intake: 16 oz.							

12 – 2 p.m. *Ast Hour of Power* — **Journal Time for Activation**

	15	16	17	18	19	20	21
Liquid Lunch (Freshly Pressed Green Juice)							
Solid Vegan Lunch							
Meditation							
Drink Water Intake: 16 oz.							

You might not complete every item every day.
These checklists serve as a guide, an invitation to complete the
practices that resonate and will help you along
your journey to healing and revitalization.

DAY	15	16	17	18	19	20	21
4 – 6 p.m. *Het-Heru Hour of Power* — **Journal Time for Inner Reflection**							
Liquid Dinner							
Solid Vegan Dinner							
Home Detox							
Drink Water Intake: 16 oz.							
8 – 10 p.m. *Nut Hour of Power* — **Journal Time for Rest**							
Healing Bath [+]							
Clay Application [++]							
Drink Water Intake: 16 oz.							
Inversion (Elevate Legs on 3 Pillows)							
Bed Rest							

[+] FOR 30 MINUTES, SOAK IN BATH WITH EPSOM OR DEAD SEA SALT.

[++] APPLY WITH GAUZE; KEEP ON OVERNIGHT.

DAYS 15–21

SACRED FOOD HEALING AFFIRMATION:

I Am a Nature Woman

Sacred Spirit, help me to break my food
addictions that cause me dis-ease. Help me to avoid
eating foods that cause cancer, high blood pressure,
tumors, anxiety, and premature aging. Help me
discern foods that are positive and contribute to my
performing positive, creative actions from foods that
are toxic and contribute to toxicity in my life. Give
me the power to eat foods that build my body into
a temple of Wellness that radiates health. May I be
so blessed to be of the mind to feed my body temple
meatless, vegetarian, fruitarian foods made for
a Sacred Body Temple. May my debilitated taste
buds be transformed into a state of purity that
I may take pleasure and delight in eating foods that
your Divine Spirit has provided for my healing.
May I find joy in consuming sacred organic fruits,
vegetables, nuts, whole grains, sprouts, and water,
all to make me into a Holy Light Being,
a Sacred Woman.

Gateway 2: Sacred Food

"On my journey to whole food organic from the garden."

DAY 15
Sacred Food Medicine Day

4 – 6 a.m. Nebt-Het Hour — Journal Time for Channeling Your Inner Vision

_____

_____

12 – 2 p.m. Ast Hour — Journal Time for Activation

_____

_____

4 – 6 p.m. Het-Heru Hour — Journal Time for Inner Reflection

_____

_____

8 – 10 p.m. Nut Hour — Journal Time for Rest

_____

_____

Gateway 2: Sacred Food

"On my journey to whole food organic from the garden."

DAY 16
Sacred Food Medicine Day

4 – 6 a.m. Nebt-Het Hour — Journal Time for Channeling Your Inner Vision

---

---

12 – 2 p.m. Ast Hour — Journal Time for Activation

---

4 – 6 p.m. Het-Heru Hour — Journal Time for Inner Reflection

---

8 – 10 p.m. Nut Hour — Journal Time for Rest

Gateway 2: Sacred Food

"On my journey to whole food organic from the garden."

DAY 17
Sacred Food Medicine Day

4 – 6 a.m. Nebt-Het Hour—Journal Time for Channeling Your Inner Vision

_____

_____

12 – 2 p.m. Ast Hour—Journal Time for Activation

_____

_____

4 – 6 p.m. Het-Heru Hour—Journal Time for Inner Reflection

_____

_____

8 – 10 p.m. Nut Hour—Journal Time for Rest

_____

_____

Gateway 2: Sacred Food

"On my journey to whole food organic from the garden."

DAY 18
Sacred Food Medicine Day

4 – 6 a.m. Nebt-Het Hour — Journal Time for Channeling Your Inner Vision

_____

_____

12 – 2 p.m. Ast Hour — Journal Time for Activation

_____

_____

4 – 6 p.m. Het-Heru Hour — Journal Time for Inner Reflection

_____

_____

8 – 10 p.m. Nut Hour — Journal Time for Rest

_____

_____

Gateway 2: Sacred Food

"On my journey to whole food organic from the garden."

DAY 19
Sacred Food Medicine Day

4 – 6 a.m. Nebt-Het Hour — Journal Time for Channeling Your Inner Vision

12 – 2 p.m. Ast Hour — Journal Time for Activation

4 – 6 p.m. Het-Heru Hour — Journal Time for Inner Reflection

8 – 10 p.m. Nut Hour — Journal Time for Rest

Gateway 2: Sacred Food

"On my journey to whole food organic from the garden."

DAY 20
Sacred Food Medicine Day

4 – 6 a.m. Nebt-Het Hour — Journal Time for Channeling Your Inner Vision

12 – 2 p.m. Ast Hour — Journal Time for Activation

4 – 6 p.m. Het-Heru Hour — Journal Time for Inner Reflection

8 – 10 p.m. Nut Hour — Journal Time for Rest

Gateway 2: Sacred Food

"On my journey to whole food organic from the garden."

DAY 21
Sacred Food Medicine Day

4 – 6 a.m. Nebt-Het Hour — Journal Time for Channeling Your Inner Vision

_____

_____

12 – 2 p.m. Ast Hour — Journal Time for Activation

_____

_____

4 – 6 p.m. Het-Heru Hour — Journal Time for Inner Reflection

_____

_____

8 – 10 p.m. Nut Hour — Journal Time for Rest

_____

_____

BES CONSCIOUSNESS

DAYS 22–28

Sacred Movement Hour of Power Daily Checklist

DAY	22	23	24	25	26	27	28

4 – 6 a.m. *Nebt-Het Hour of Power* — **Journal Time for Channeling Your Inner Vision**

	22	23	24	25	26	27	28
Inversion (Elevate Legs on 3 Pillows)							
Hydrotherapy (Shower/Bath, Brush Teeth, Enema)							
Spiritual Observances 1–14 in the *Sacred Woman* Text for This Gateway							
Womb Yoga Fitness							
Liquid Breakfast (Freshly Pressed Fruit Juice)							
Solid Breakfast							
Herbal Tonic (Womb Care Love Herbal Detox Formula)							
Drink Water Intake: 16 oz.							

12 – 2 p.m. *Ast Hour of Power* — **Journal Time for Activation**

	22	23	24	25	26	27	28
Liquid Lunch (Freshly Pressed Green Juice)							
Solid Vegan Lunch							
Meditation							
Drink Water Intake: 16 oz.							

You might not complete every item every day.
These checklists serve as a guide, an invitation to complete
the practices that resonate and will help you along
your journey to healing and revitalization.

DAY	22	23	24	25	26	27	28
4 – 6 p.m. *Het-Heru Hour of Power* — Journal Time for Inner Reflection							
Liquid Dinner							
Solid Vegan Dinner							
Home Detox							
Drink Water Intake: 16 oz.							
8 – 10 p.m. *Nut Hour of Power* — Journal Time for Rest							
Healing Bath +							
Clay Application + +							
Drink Water Intake: 16 oz.							
Inversion (Elevate Legs on 3 Pillows)							
Bed Rest							

+ FOR 30 MINUTES, SOAK IN BATH WITH EPSOM OR DEAD SEA SALT.

++ APPLY WITH GAUZE; KEEP ON OVERNIGHT.

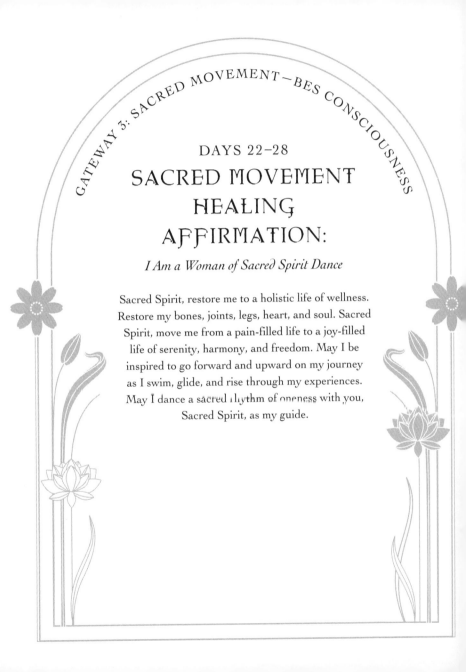

DAYS 22–28

SACRED MOVEMENT HEALING AFFIRMATION:

I Am a Woman of Sacred Spirit Dance

Sacred Spirit, restore me to a holistic life of wellness.
Restore my bones, joints, legs, heart, and soul. Sacred
Spirit, move me from a pain-filled life to a joy-filled
life of serenity, harmony, and freedom. May I be
inspired to go forward and upward on my journey
as I swim, glide, and rise through my experiences.
May I dance a sacred rhythm of oneness with you,
Sacred Spirit, as my guide.

Gateway 3: Sacred Movement

"I am that I am on my journey to freedom through
  moving forward."

DAY 22
Sacred Movement Medicine Day

4 – 6 a.m. Nebt-Het Hour — Journal Time for Channeling Your Inner Vision

12 – 2 p.m. Ast Hour — Journal Time for Activation

4 – 6 p.m. Het-Heru Hour — Journal Time for Inner Reflection

8 – 10 p.m. Nut Hour — Journal Time for Rest

Gateway 3: Sacred Movement

"I am that I am on my journey to freedom through
 moving forward."

DAY 23
Sacred Movement Medicine Day

4 – 6 a.m. Nebt-Het Hour — Journal Time for Channeling Your Inner Vision

_____

_____

12 – 2 p.m. Ast Hour — Journal Time for Activation

_____

_____

4 – 6 p.m. Het-Heru Hour — Journal Time for Inner Reflection

_____

_____

8 – 10 p.m. Nut Hour — Journal Time for Rest

_____

_____

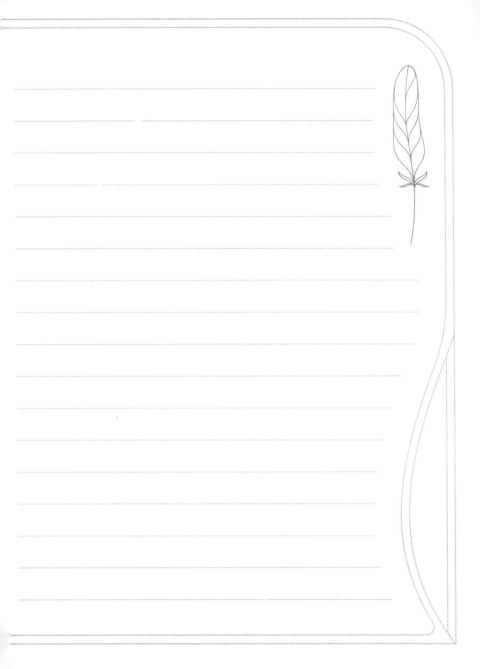

Gateway 3: Sacred Movement

"I am that I am on my journey to freedom through
moving forward."

DAY 24
Sacred Movement Medicine Day

4 – 6 a.m. Nebt-Het Hour — Journal Time for Channeling Your Inner Vision

12 – 2 p.m. Ast Hour — Journal Time for Activation

4 – 6 p.m. Het-Heru Hour — Journal Time for Inner Reflection

8 – 10 p.m. Nut Hour — Journal Time for Rest

Gateway 3: Sacred Movement

"I am that I am on my journey to freedom through moving forward."

DAY 25
Sacred Movement Medicine Day

4 – 6 a.m. Nebt-Het Hour — Journal Time for Channeling Your Inner Vision

12 – 2 p.m. Ast Hour — Journal Time for Activation

4 – 6 p.m. Het-Heru Hour — Journal Time for Inner Reflection

8 – 10 p.m. Nut Hour — Journal Time for Rest

Gateway 3: Sacred Movement

"I am that I am on my journey to freedom through
 moving forward."

DAY 26
Sacred Movement Medicine Day

4 – 6 a.m. Nebt-Het Hour—Journal Time for Channeling Your Inner Vision

_____

_____

12 – 2 p.m. Ast Hour—Journal Time for Activation

_____

_____

4 – 6 p.m. Het-Heru Hour—Journal Time for Inner Reflection

_____

_____

8 – 10 p.m. Nut Hour—Journal Time for Rest

_____

_____

Gateway 3: Sacred Movement

"I am that I am on my journey to freedom through moving forward."

DAY 27
Sacred Movement Medicine Day

4 – 6 a.m. Nebt-Het Hour — Journal Time for Channeling Your Inner Vision

12 – 2 p.m. Ast Hour — Journal Time for Activation

4 – 6 p.m. Het-Heru Hour — Journal Time for Inner Reflection

8 – 10 p.m. Nut Hour — Journal Time for Rest

Gateway 3: Sacred Movement

"I am that I am on my journey to freedom through moving forward."

DAY 28
Sacred Movement Medicine Day

4 – 6 a.m. Nebt-Het Hour — Journal Time for Channeling Your Inner Vision

_____

_____

12 – 2 p.m. Ast Hour — Journal Time for Activation

_____

_____

4 – 6 p.m. Het-Heru Hour — Journal Time for Inner Reflection

_____

_____

8 – 10 p.m. Nut Hour — Journal Time for Rest

_____

_____

GATEWAY 4: SACRED BEAUTY

HET-HERU CONSCIOUSNESS

DAYS 29–35

Sacred Beauty Hour of Power Daily Checklist

DAY	29	30	31	32	33	34	35
4 – 6 a.m. *Nebt-Het Hour of Power* — Journal Time for Channeling Your Inner Vision							
Inversion (Elevate Legs on 3 Pillows)							
Hydrotherapy (Shower/Bath, Brush Teeth, Enema)							
Spiritual Observances 1–14 in the *Sacred Woman* Text for This Gateway							
Womb Yoga Fitness							
Liquid Breakfast (Freshly Pressed Fruit Juice)							
Solid Breakfast							
Herbal Tonic (Womb Care Love Herbal Detox Formula)							
Drink Water Intake: 16 oz.							

12 – 2 p.m. *Ast Hour of Power* — Journal Time for Activation

	29	30	31	32	33	34	35
Liquid Lunch (Freshly Pressed Green Juice)							
Solid Vegan Lunch							
Meditation							
Drink Water Intake: 16 oz.							

You might not complete every item every day.
These checklists serve as a guide, an invitation to complete
the practices that resonate and will help you along
your journey to healing and revitalization.

DAY	29	30	31	32	33	34	35

4 – 6 p.m. *Het-Heru Hour of Power* — Journal Time for Inner Reflection

Liquid Dinner							
Solid Vegan Dinner							
Home Detox							
Drink Water Intake: 16 oz.							

8 – 10 p.m. *Nut Hour of Power* — Journal Time for Rest

Healing Bath +							
Clay Application ++							
Drink Water Intake: 16 oz.							
Inversion (Elevate Legs on 3 Pillows)							
Bed Rest							

+ FOR 30 MINUTES, SOAK IN BATH WITH EPSOM OR DEAD SEA SALT.

++ APPLY WITH GAUZE; KEEP ON OVERNIGHT.

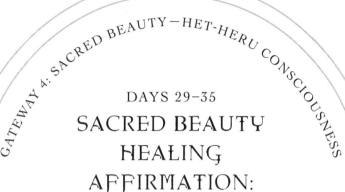

DAYS 29–35

SACRED BEAUTY HEALING AFFIRMATION:

I Am a Woman of Grace

Sacred Spirit, restore the beauty in my mind, my heart, and my soul. May my inner child radiate beauty and peace, that through me I may evolve into a whole woman. May my body temple be like that of a Sacred Altar, so that I may maintain a beautiful spirit, dressed in an array of rainbow colors, reflecting the beauty and the boundless creativity of your light. May divine beauty reflect in my thoughts, and may the attitudes that reflect my consciousness create the sacredness of my dress. May I be a walking embodiment of the beauty of the Creator, that others may be lifted as I emanate Sacred Beauty in all my ways.

Gateway 4: Sacred Beauty

"I am that I am on my journey to my inner and outer beauty."

DAY 29
Sacred Beauty Medicine Day

4 – 6 a.m. Nebt-Het Hour — Journal Time for Channeling Your Inner Vision

_____

_____

12 – 2 p.m. Ast Hour — Journal Time for Activation

_____

_____

4 – 6 p.m. Het-Heru Hour — Journal Time for Inner Reflection

_____

_____

8 – 10 p.m. Nut Hour — Journal Time for Rest

_____

_____

Gateway 4: Sacred Beauty

"I am that I am on my journey to my inner and outer beauty."

DAY 30
Sacred Beauty Medicine Day

4 – 6 a.m. Nebt-Het Hour — Journal Time for Channeling Your Inner Vision

12 – 2 p.m. Ast Hour — Journal Time for Activation

4 – 6 p.m. Het-Heru Hour — Journal Time for Inner Reflection

8 – 10 p.m. Nut Hour — Journal Time for Rest

Gateway 4: Sacred Beauty

"I am that I am on my journey to my inner and outer beauty."

DAY 31
Sacred Beauty Medicine Day

4 – 6 a.m. Nebt-Het Hour — Journal Time for Channeling Your Inner Vision

---

---

12 – 2 p.m. Ast Hour — Journal Time for Activation

---

4 – 6 p.m. Het-Heru Hour — Journal Time for Inner Reflection

---

8 – 10 p.m. Nut Hour — Journal Time for Rest

Gateway 4: Sacred Beauty

"I am that I am on my journey to my inner and outer beauty."

DAY 32
Sacred Beauty Medicine Day

4 – 6 a.m. Nebt-Het Hour — Journal Time for Channeling Your Inner Vision

_____

_____

12 – 2 p.m. Ast Hour — Journal Time for Activation

_____

_____

4 – 6 p.m. Het-Heru Hour — Journal Time for Inner Reflection

_____

_____

8 – 10 p.m. Nut Hour — Journal Time for Rest

_____

_____

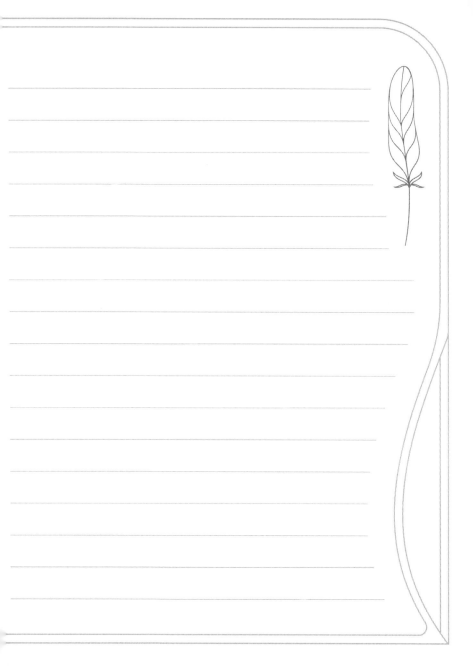

Gateway 4: Sacred Beauty

"I am that I am on my journey to my inner and outer beauty."

DAY 33
Sacred Beauty Medicine Day

4 – 6 a.m. Nebt-Het Hour — Journal Time for Channeling Your Inner Vision

12 – 2 p.m. Ast Hour — Journal Time for Activation

4 – 6 p.m. Het-Heru Hour — Journal Time for Inner Reflection

8 – 10 p.m. Nut Hour — Journal Time for Rest

Gateway 4: Sacred Beauty

"I am that I am on my journey to my inner and outer beauty."

DAY 34
Sacred Beauty Medicine Day

4 – 6 a.m. Nebt-Het Hour — Journal Time for Channeling Your Inner Vision

12 – 2 p.m. Ast Hour — Journal Time for Activation

4 – 6 p.m. Het-Heru Hour — Journal Time for Inner Reflection

8 – 10 p.m. Nut Hour — Journal Time for Rest

Gateway 4: Sacred Beauty

"I am that I am on my journey to my inner and outer beauty."

DAY 35
Sacred Beauty Medicine Day

4 – 6 a.m. Nebt-Het Hour — Journal Time for Channeling Your Inner Vision

12 – 2 p.m. Ast Hour — Journal Time for Activation

4 – 6 p.m. Het-Heru Hour — Journal Time for Inner Reflection

8 – 10 p.m. Nut Hour — Journal Time for Rest

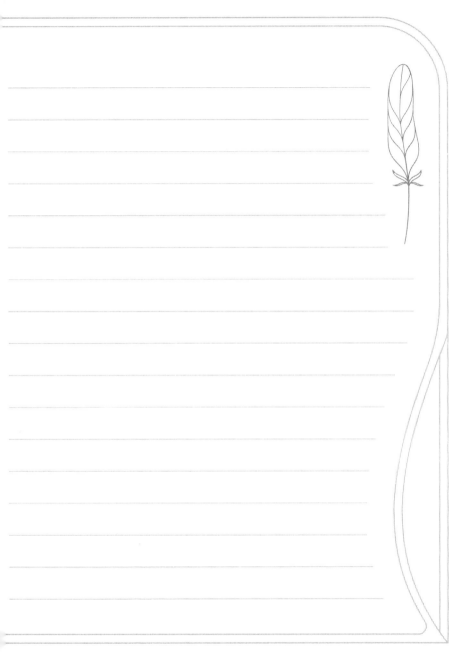

NEBT-HET CONSCIOUSNESS

DAYS 36–42

Sacred Space Hour of Power Daily Checklist

DAY	36	37	38	39	40	41	42
4 – 6 a.m. *Nebt-Het Hour of Power* **– Journal Time for Channeling Your Inner Vision**							
Inversion (Elevate Legs on 3 Pillows)							
Hydrotherapy (Shower/Bath, Brush Teeth, Enema)							
Spiritual Observances 1–14 in the *Sacred Woman* Text for This Gateway							
Womb Yoga Fitness							
Liquid Breakfast (Freshly Pressed Fruit Juice)							
Solid Breakfast							
Herbal Tonic (Womb Care Love Herbal Detox Formula)							
Drink Water Intake: 16 oz.							

12 – 2 p.m. *Ast Hour of Power* **– Journal Time for Activation**

	36	37	38	39	40	41	42
Liquid Lunch (Freshly Pressed Green Juice)							
Solid Vegan Lunch							
Meditation							
Drink Water Intake: 16 oz.							

You might not complete every item every day.
These checklists serve as a guide, an invitation to the
practices that resonate and will help you along
your journey to healing and revitalization.

DAY	36	37	38	39	40	41	42

4 – 6 p.m. *Het-Heru Hour of Power* — Journal Time for Inner Reflection

	36	37	38	39	40	41	42
Liquid Dinner							
Solid Vegan Dinner							
Home Detox							
Drink Water Intake: 16 oz.							

8 – 10 p.m. *Nut Hour of Power* — Journal Time for Rest

Healing Bath +							
Clay Application ++							
Drink Water Intake: 16 oz.							
Inversion (Elevate Legs on 3 Pillows)							
Bed Rest							

+ FOR 30 MINUTES, SOAK IN BATH WITH EPSOM OR DEAD SEA SALT.

++ APPLY WITH GAUZE; KEEP ON OVERNIGHT.

DAYS 36–42

SACRED SPACE HEALING AFFIRMATION:

I Am a Woman of Intuitive Skill

Sacred Spirit, restore my Sacred Space. Assist me
in keeping my inner and outer spaces sacred and
clean, whether the space is in my body, my home,
or my office and whether I am at work or at play.
May all the space in me and around me be
free of clutter, confusion, and dismay. May my
environment be as pure, open, and in Divine Order
as the sky, ocean, and sun. May my environment be
in Divine Order as the planet Earth was in its first
days, when the world was clean and whole. May
we respect nature, our environment, and our space.
May we return to purity as it was in the beginning.
May my space always emanate peace and serenity.
May my intuition that resides in my Sacred Space
be clear, that I may walk in alignment with you,
Divine Sacred Spirit. Today, I deem my space
a Sacred Space.

Gateway 5: Sacred Space

"I am trusting the power of my intuition with each day gone by."

DAY 36
Sacred Space Medicine Day

4 – 6 a.m. Nebt-Het Hour — Journal Time for Channeling Your Inner Vision

---

---

12 – 2 p.m. Ast Hour — Journal Time for Activation

---

4 – 6 p.m. Het-Heru Hour — Journal Time for Inner Reflection

---

8 – 10 p.m. Nut Hour — Journal Time for Rest

Gateway 5: Sacred Space

"I am trusting the power of my intuition with each day gone by."

DAY 37
Sacred Space Medicine Day

4 – 6 a.m. Nebt-Het Hour — Journal Time for Channeling Your Inner Vision

12 – 2 p.m. Ast Hour — Journal Time for Activation

4 – 6 p.m. Het-Heru Hour — Journal Time for Inner Reflection

8 – 10 p.m. Nut Hour — Journal Time for Rest

Gateway 5: Sacred Space

"I am trusting the power of my intuition with each day gone by."

DAY 38
Sacred Space Medicine Day

4 – 6 a.m. Nebt-Het Hour—Journal Time for Channeling Your Inner Vision

_____

_____

12 – 2 p.m. Ast Hour—Journal Time for Activation

_____

_____

4 – 6 p.m. Het-Heru Hour—Journal Time for Inner Reflection

_____

_____

8 – 10 p.m. Nut Hour—Journal Time for Rest

_____

_____

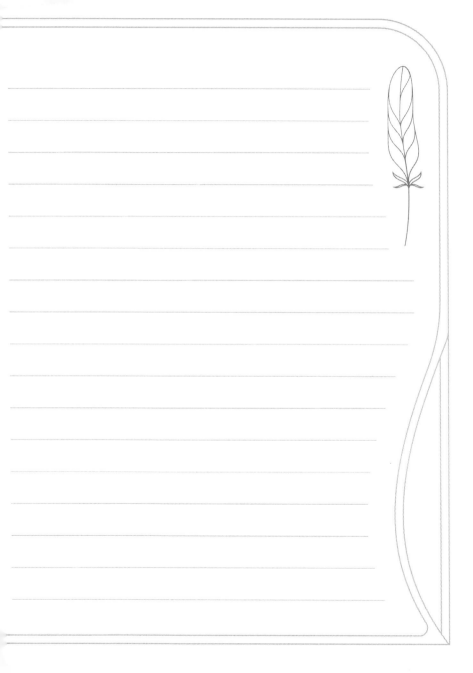

Gateway 5: Sacred Space

"I am trusting the power of my intuition with each day gone by."

DAY 39
Sacred Space Medicine Day

4 – 6 a.m. Nebt-Het Hour — Journal Time for Channeling Your Inner Vision

12 – 2 p.m. Ast Hour — Journal Time for Activation

4 – 6 p.m. Het-Heru Hour — Journal Time for Inner Reflection

8 – 10 p.m. Nut Hour — Journal Time for Rest

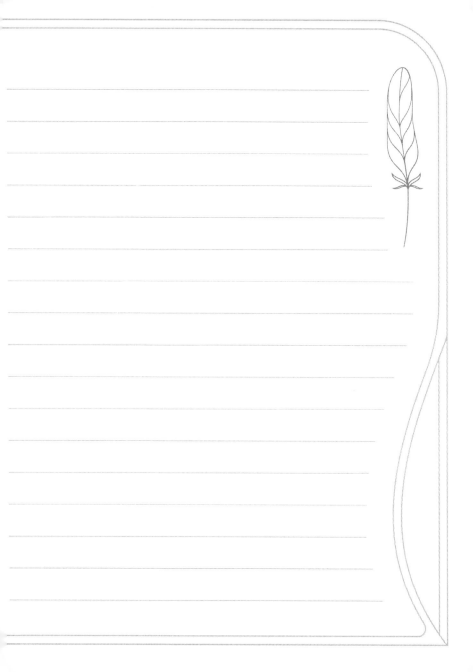

Gateway 5: Sacred Space

"I am trusting the power of my intuition with each day gone by."

DAY 40
Sacred Space Medicine Day

4 – 6 a.m. Nebt-Het Hour — Journal Time for Channeling Your Inner Vision

12 – 2 p.m. Ast Hour — Journal Time for Activation

4 – 6 p.m. Het-Heru Hour — Journal Time for Inner Reflection

8 – 10 p.m. Nut Hour — Journal Time for Rest

Gateway 5: Sacred Space

"I am trusting the power of my intuition with each day gone by."

DAY 41
Sacred Space Medicine Day

4 – 6 a.m. Nebt-Het Hour — Journal Time for Channeling Your Inner Vision

_____

_____

12 – 2 p.m. Ast Hour — Journal Time for Activation

_____

_____

4 – 6 p.m. Het-Heru Hour — Journal Time for Inner Reflection

_____

_____

8 – 10 p.m. Nut Hour — Journal Time for Rest

_____

_____

Gateway 5: Sacred Space

"I am trusting the power of my intuition with each day gone by."

DAY 42
Sacred Space Medicine Day

4 – 6 a.m. Nebt-Het Hour—Journal Time for Channeling Your Inner Vision

_____

_____

12 – 2 p.m. Ast Hour—Journal Time for Activation

_____

_____

4 – 6 p.m. Het-Heru Hour—Journal Time for Inner Reflection

_____

_____

8 – 10 p.m. Nut Hour—Journal Time for Rest

_____

_____

GATEWAY 6: SACRED HEALING
SEKHMET CONSCIOUSNESS

DAYS 43–49

Sacred Healing Hour of Power Daily Checklist

DAY	43	44	45	46	47	48	49

4 – 6 a.m. *Nebt-Het Hour of Power* — Journal Time for Channeling Your Inner Vision

	43	44	45	46	47	48	49
Inversion (Elevate Legs on 3 Pillows)							
Hydrotherapy (Shower/Bath, Brush Teeth, Enema)							
Spiritual Observances 1–14 in the *Sacred Woman* Text for This Gateway							
Womb Yoga Fitness							
Liquid Breakfast (Freshly Pressed Fruit Juice)							
Solid Breakfast							
Herbal Tonic (Womb Care Love Herbal Detox Formula)							
Drink Water Intake: 16 oz.							

12 – 2 p.m. *Ast Hour of Power* — Journal Time for Activation

	43	44	45	46	47	48	49
Liquid Lunch (Freshly Pressed Green Juice)							
Solid Vegan Lunch							
Meditation							
Drink Water Intake: 16 oz.							

You might not complete every item every day.
These checklists serve as a guide, an invitation to complete
the practices that resonate and will help you along
your journey to healing and revitalization.

DAY	43	44	45	46	47	48	49
4 – 6 p.m. *Het-Heru Hour of Power* — Journal Time for Inner Reflection							
Liquid Dinner							
Solid Vegan Dinner							
Home Detox							
Drink Water Intake: 16 oz.							
8 – 10 p.m. *Nut Hour of Power* — Journal Time for Rest							
Healing Bath ✝							
Clay Application ✝✝							
Drink Water Intake: 16 oz.							
Inversion (Elevate Legs on 3 Pillows)							
Bed Rest							

✝ FOR 30 MINUTES, SOAK IN BATH WITH EPSOM OR DEAD SEA SALT.

✝✝ APPLY WITH GAUZE; KEEP ON OVERNIGHT.

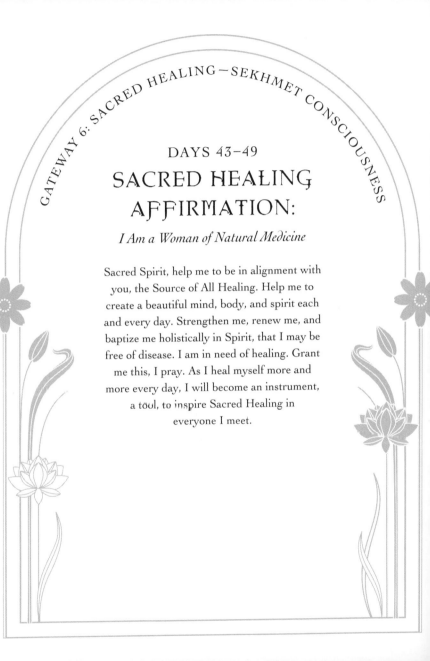

DAYS 43–49

SACRED HEALING

AFFIRMATION:

I Am a Woman of Natural Medicine

Sacred Spirit, help me to be in alignment with
you, the Source of All Healing. Help me to
create a beautiful mind, body, and spirit each
and every day. Strengthen me, renew me, and
baptize me holistically in Spirit, that I may be
free of disease. I am in need of healing. Grant
me this, I pray. As I heal myself more and
more every day, I will become an instrument,
a tool, to inspire Sacred Healing in
everyone I meet.

Gateway 6: Sacred Healing

"I am a healer and I can heal myself."

DAY 43
Sacred Healing Medicine Day

4 – 6 a.m. Nebt-Het Hour — Journal Time for Channeling Your Inner Vision

12 – 2 p.m. Ast Hour — Journal Time for Activation

4 – 6 p.m. Het-Heru Hour — Journal Time for Inner Reflection

8 – 10 p.m. Nut Hour — Journal Time for Rest

Gateway 6: Sacred Healing

"I am a healer and I can heal myself."

DAY 44
Sacred Healing Medicine Day

4 – 6 a.m. Nebt-Het Hour — Journal Time for Channeling Your Inner Vision

_____

_____

12 – 2 p.m. Ast Hour — Journal Time for Activation

_____

_____

4 – 6 p.m. Het-Heru Hour — Journal Time for Inner Reflection

_____

_____

8 – 10 p.m. Nut Hour — Journal Time for Rest

_____

_____

Gateway 6: Sacred Healing

"I am a healer and I can heal myself."

DAY 45
Sacred Healing Medicine Day

4 – 6 a.m. Nebt-Het Hour — Journal Time for Channeling Your Inner Vision

_____

_____

12 – 2 p.m. Ast Hour — Journal Time for Activation

_____

_____

4 – 6 p.m. Het-Heru Hour — Journal Time for Inner Reflection

_____

_____

8 – 10 p.m. Nut Hour — Journal Time for Rest

_____

_____

Gateway 6: Sacred Healing

"I am a healer and I can heal myself."

DAY 46
Sacred Healing Medicine Day

4 – 6 a.m. Nebt-Het Hour — Journal Time for Channeling Your Inner Vision

---

---

12 – 2 p.m. Ast Hour — Journal Time for Activation

---

4 – 6 p.m. Het-Heru Hour — Journal Time for Inner Reflection

---

8 – 10 p.m. Nut Hour — Journal Time for Rest

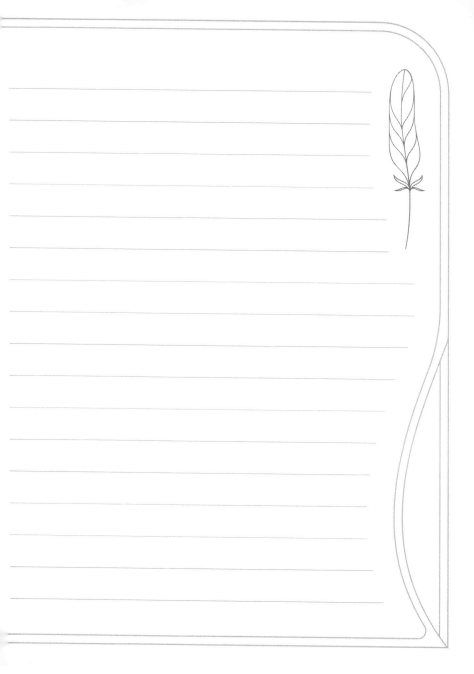

Gateway 6: Sacred Healing

"I am a healer and I can heal myself."

DAY 47
Sacred Healing Medicine Day

4 – 6 a.m. Nebt-Het Hour — Journal Time for Channeling Your Inner Vision

12 – 2 p.m. Ast Hour — Journal Time for Activation

4 – 6 p.m. Het-Heru Hour — Journal Time for Inner Reflection

8 – 10 p.m. Nut Hour — Journal Time for Rest

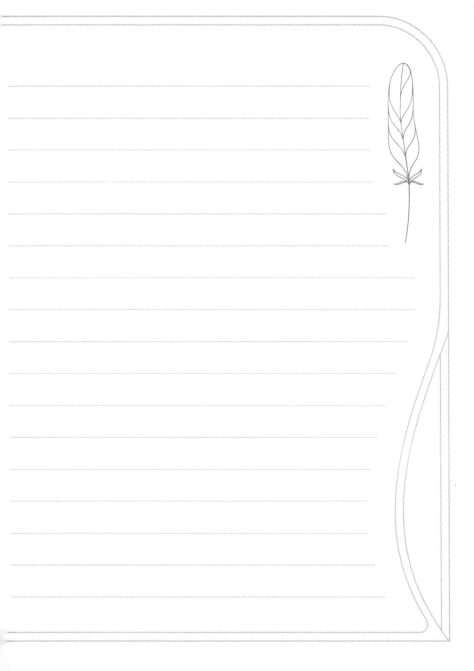

Gateway 6: Sacred Healing

"I am a healer and I can heal myself."

DAY 48
Sacred Healing Medicine Day

4 – 6 a.m. Nebt-Het Hour — Journal Time for Channeling Your Inner Vision

---

---

12 – 2 p.m. Ast Hour — Journal Time for Activation

---

4 – 6 p.m. Het-Heru Hour — Journal Time for Inner Reflection

---

8 – 10 p.m. Nut Hour — Journal Time for Rest

Gateway 6: Sacred Healing

"I am a healer and I can heal myself."

DAY 49
Sacred Healing Medicine Day

4 – 6 a.m. Nebt-Het Hour — Journal Time for Channeling Your Inner Vision

12 – 2 p.m. Ast Hour — Journal Time for Activation

4 – 6 p.m. Het-Heru Hour — Journal Time for Inner Reflection

8 – 10 p.m. Nut Hour — Journal Time for Rest

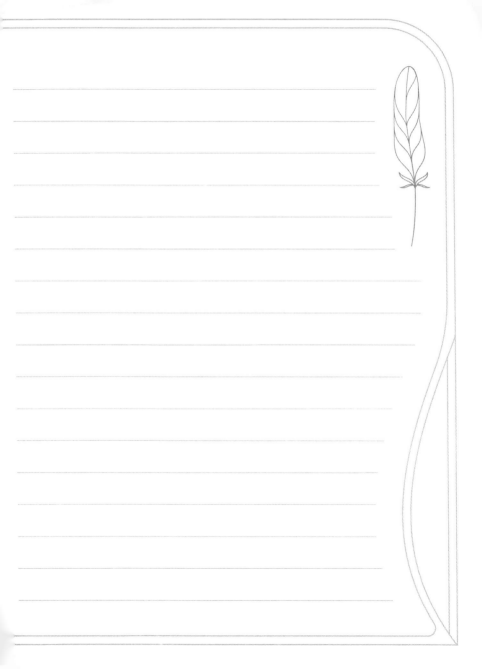

MAAT CONSCIOUSNESS

DAYS 50–56

Sacred Relationships Hour of Power Daily Checklist

DAY	50	51	52	53	54	55	56

4 – 6 a.m. *Nebt-Het Hour of Power* — Journal Time for Channeling Your Inner Vision

	50	51	52	53	54	55	56
Inversion (Elevate Legs on 3 Pillows)							
Hydrotherapy (Shower/Bath, Brush Teeth, Enema)							
Spiritual Observances 1–14 in the *Sacred Woman* Text for This Gateway							
Womb Yoga Fitness							
Liquid Breakfast (Freshly Pressed Fruit Juice)							
Solid Breakfast							
Herbal Tonic (Womb Care Love Herbal Detox Formula)							
Drink Intake: 16 oz.							

12 – 2 p.m. *Ast Hour of Power* — Journal Time for Activation

	50	51	52	53	54	55	56
Liquid Lunch (Freshly Pressed Green Juice)							
Solid Vegan Lunch							
Meditation							
Drink Water Intake: 16 oz.							

You might not complete every item every day.
These checklists serve as a guide, an invitation to complete
the practices that resonate and will help you along
your journey to healing and revitalization.

DAY	50	51	52	53	54	55	56

4 – 6 p.m. *Het-Heru Hour of Power* — Journal Time for Inner Reflection

	50	51	52	53	54	55	56
Liquid Dinner							
Solid Vegan Dinner							
Home Detox							
Drink Water Intake: 16 oz.							

8 – 10 p.m. *Nut Hour of Power* — Journal Time for Rest

	50	51	52	53	54	55	56
Healing Bath +							
Clay Application ++							
Drink Water Intake: 16 oz.							
Inversion (Elevate Legs on 3 Pillows)							
Bed Rest							

+ FOR 30 MINUTES, SOAK IN BATH WITH EPSOM OR DEAD SEA SALT.

++ APPLY WITH GAUZE; KEEP ON OVERNIGHT.

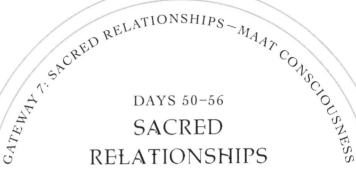

DAYS 50–56

SACRED RELATIONSHIPS HEALING AFFIRMATION:

I Am a Woman of Harmony and Balance

Sacred Spirit, I stand in need of Sacred
Relationships in my life. Sacred Spirit, may
I create a Sacred Relationship with you and
with all my relations. Help me to attract
and establish harmonious, wholesome, and
healthy relationships. Help me to unblock
and release old hurt feelings, resentments,
and hostility trapped within my body temple.
Help me to have the vision and the strength
to learn from all my relationships, as they
are all my reflections and have value in my
life. As I reflect on the lessons and insight
provided by my relationships, I give thanks
to the Divine in me and in all others.

Gateway 7: Sacred Relationships

"I am a reflection of all my relationships.
As I heal myself, I heal my relations."

DAY 50
Sacred Relationships Medicine Day

4 – 6 a.m. Nebt-Het Hour — Journal Time for Channeling Your Inner Vision

12 – 2 p.m. Ast Hour — Journal Time for Activation

4 – 6 p.m. Het-Heru Hour — Journal Time for Inner Reflection

8 – 10 p.m. Nut Hour — Journal Time for Rest

Gateway 7: Sacred Relationships

"I am a reflection of all my relationships.
As I heal myself, I heal my relations."

DAY 51
Sacred Relationships Medicine Day

4 – 6 a.m. Nebt-Het Hour — Journal Time for Channeling Your Inner Vision

12 – 2 p.m. Ast Hour — Journal Time for Activation

4 – 6 p.m. Het-Heru Hour — Journal Time for Inner Reflection

8 – 10 p.m. Nut Hour — Journal Time for Rest

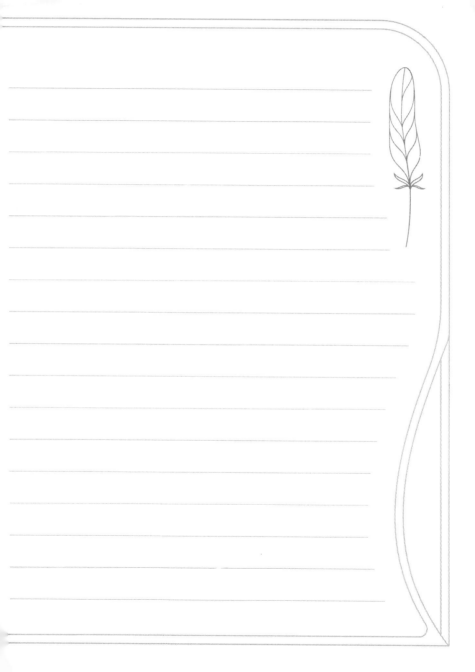

Gateway 7: Sacred Relationships

"I am a reflection of all my relationships.
As I heal myself, I heal my relations."

DAY 52
Sacred Relationships Medicine Day

4 – 6 a.m. Nebt-Het Hour — Journal Time for Channeling Your Inner Vision

12 – 2 p.m. Ast Hour — Journal Time for Activation

4 – 6 p.m. Het-Heru Hour — Journal Time for Inner Reflection

8 – 10 p.m. Nut Hour — Journal Time for Rest

Gateway 7: Sacred Relationships

"I am a reflection of all my relationships.
As I heal myself, I heal my relations."

DAY 53
Sacred Relationships Medicine Day

4 – 6 a.m. Nebt-Het Hour—Journal Time for Channeling Your Inner Vision

12 – 2 p.m. Ast Hour—Journal Time for Activation

4 – 6 p.m. Het-Heru Hour—Journal Time for Inner Reflection

8 – 10 p.m. Nut Hour—Journal Time for Rest

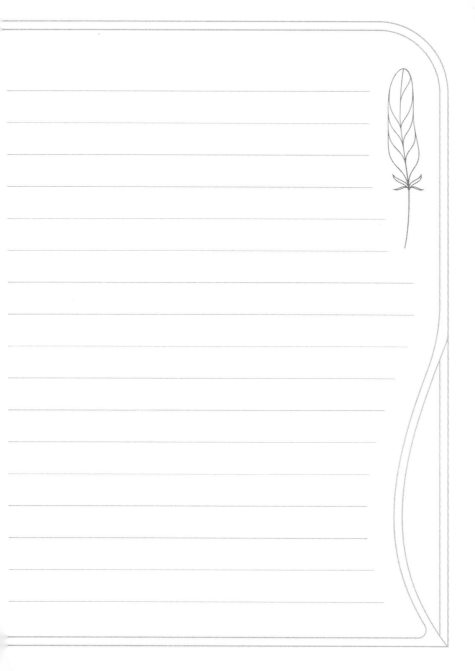

Gateway 7: Sacred Relationships

"I am a reflection of all my relationships.
As I heal myself, I heal my relations."

DAY 54
Sacred Relationships Medicine Day

4 – 6 a.m. Nebt-Het Hour — Journal Time for Channeling Your Inner Vision

12 – 2 p.m. Ast Hour — Journal Time for Activation

4 – 6 p.m. Het-Heru Hour — Journal Time for Inner Reflection

8 – 10 p.m. Nut Hour — Journal Time for Rest

Gateway 7: Sacred Relationships

"I am a reflection of all my relationships.
As I heal myself, I heal my relations."

DAY 55
Sacred Relationships Medicine Day

4 – 6 a.m. Nebt-Het Hour—Journal Time for Channeling Your Inner Vision

_____

_____

12 – 2 p.m. Ast Hour—Journal Time for Activation

_____

_____

4 – 6 p.m. Het-Heru Hour—Journal Time for Inner Reflection

_____

_____

8 – 10 p.m. Nut Hour—Journal Time for Rest

_____

_____

Gateway 7: Sacred Relationships

"I am a reflection of all my relationships.
As I heal myself, I heal my relations."

DAY 56
Sacred Relationships Medicine Day

4 – 6 a.m. Nebt-Het Hour—Journal Time for Channeling Your Inner Vision

12 – 2 p.m. Ast Hour—Journal Time for Activation

4 – 6 p.m. Het-Heru Hour—Journal Time for Inner Reflection

8 – 10 p.m. Nut Hour—Journal Time for Rest

AST CONSCIOUSNESS

DAYS 57–63

Sacred Union Hour of Power Daily Checklist

DAY	57	58	59	60	61	62	63
4 – 6 a.m. *Nebt-Het Hour of Power*— Journal Time for Channeling Your Inner Vision							
Inversion (Elevate Legs on 3 Pillows)							
Hydrotherapy (Shower/Bath, Brush Teeth, Enema)							
Spiritual Observances 1–14 in the *Sacred Woman* Text for This Gateway							
Womb Yoga Fitness							
Liquid Breakfast (Freshly Pressed Fruit Juice)							
Solid Breakfast							
Herbal Tonic (Womb Care Love Herbal Detox Formula)							
Drink Water Intake: 16 oz.							

12 – 2 p.m. *Ast Hour of Power*— Journal Time for Activation

	57	58	59	60	61	62	63
Liquid Lunch (Freshly Pressed Green Juice)							
Solid Vegan Lunch							
Meditation							
Drink Water Intake: 16 oz.							

You might not complete every item every day.
These checklists serve as a guide, an invitation to complete the
practices that resonate and will help you along
your journey to healing and revitalization.

DAY	57	58	59	60	61	62	63
4 – 6 p.m. *Het-Heru Hour of Power* — Journal Time for Inner Reflection							
Liquid Dinner							
Solid Vegan Dinner							
Home Detox							
Drink Water Intake: 16 oz.							
8 – 10 p.m. *Nut Hour of Power* — Journal Time for Rest							
Healing Bath +							
Clay Application ++							
Drink Water Intake: 16 oz.							
Inversion (Elevate Legs on 3 Pillows)							
Bed Rest							

+ FOR 30 MINUTES, SOAK IN BATH WITH EPSOM OR DEAD SEA SALT.

++ APPLY WITH GAUZE; KEEP ON OVERNIGHT.

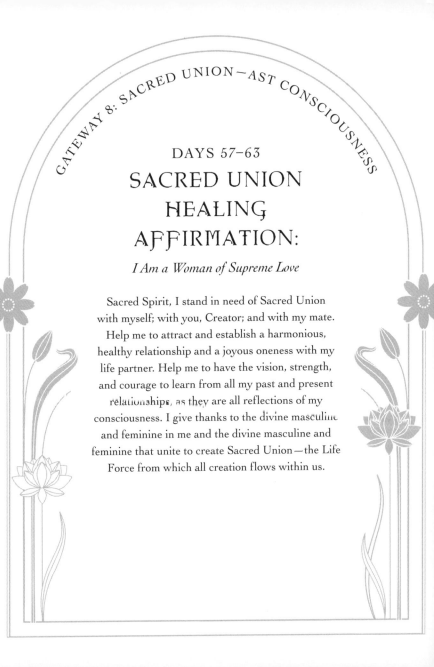

DAYS 57–63

SACRED UNION HEALING AFFIRMATION:

I Am a Woman of Supreme Love

Sacred Spirit, I stand in need of Sacred Union
with myself; with you, Creator; and with my mate.
Help me to attract and establish a harmonious,
healthy relationship and a joyous oneness with my
life partner. Help me to have the vision, strength,
and courage to learn from all my past and present
relationships, as they are all reflections of my
consciousness. I give thanks to the divine masculine
and feminine in me and the divine masculine and
feminine that unite to create Sacred Union—the Life
Force from which all creation flows within us.

Gateway 8: Sacred Union

"I am that I am sitting on my seat of power, causing me
to be in Sacred Union with my Divine Reflection."

DAY 57
Sacred Union Medicine Day

4 – 6 a.m. Nebt-Het Hour — Journal Time for Channeling Your Inner Vision

12 – 2 p.m. Ast Hour — Journal Time for Activation

4 – 6 p.m. Het-Heru Hour — Journal Time for Inner Reflection

8 – 10 p.m. Nut Hour — Journal Time for Rest

Gateway 8: Sacred Union

"I am that I am sitting on my seat of power, causing me
to be in Sacred Union with my Divine Reflection."

DAY 58
Sacred Union Medicine Day

4 – 6 a.m. Nebt-Het Hour — Journal Time for Channeling Your Inner Vision

12 – 2 p.m. Ast Hour — Journal Time for Activation

4 – 6 p.m. Het-Heru Hour — Journal Time for Inner Reflection

8 – 10 p.m. Nut Hour — Journal Time for Rest

Gateway 8: Sacred Union

"I am that I am sitting on my seat of power, causing me to be in Sacred Union with my Divine Reflection."

DAY 59
Sacred Union Medicine Day

4 – 6 a.m. Nebt-Het Hour — Journal Time for Channeling Your Inner Vision

12 – 2 p.m. Ast Hour — Journal Time for Activation

4 – 6 p.m. Het-Heru Hour — Journal Time for Inner Reflection

8 – 10 p.m. Nut Hour — Journal Time for Rest

Gateway 8: Sacred Union

"I am that I am sitting on my seat of power, causing me
to be in Sacred Union with my Divine Reflection."

DAY 60
Sacred Union Medicine Day

4 – 6 a.m. Nebt-Het Hour — Journal Time for Channeling Your Inner Vision

12 – 2 p.m. Ast Hour — Journal Time for Activation

4 – 6 p.m. Het-Heru Hour — Journal Time for Inner Reflection

8 – 10 p.m. Nut Hour — Journal Time for Rest

Gateway 8: Sacred Union

"I am that I am sitting on my seat of power, causing me
to be in Sacred Union with my Divine Reflection."

DAY 61
Sacred Union Medicine Day

4 – 6 a.m. Nebt-Het Hour — Journal Time for Channeling Your Inner Vision

12 – 2 p.m. Ast Hour — Journal Time for Activation

4 – 6 p.m. Het-Heru Hour — Journal Time for Inner Reflection

8 – 10 p.m. Nut Hour — Journal Time for Rest

Gateway 8: Sacred Union

"I am that I am sitting on my seat of power, causing me
to be in Sacred Union with my Divine Reflection."

DAY 62
Sacred Union Medicine Day

4 – 6 a.m. Nebt-Het Hour — Journal Time for Channeling Your Inner Vision

---

12 – 2 p.m. Ast Hour — Journal Time for Activation

---

4 – 6 p.m. Het-Heru Hour — Journal Time for Inner Reflection

---

8 – 10 p.m. Nut Hour — Journal Time for Rest

Gateway 8: Sacred Union

"I am that I am sitting on my seat of power, causing me
to be in Sacred Union with my Divine Reflection."

DAY 63
Sacred Union Medicine Day

4 – 6 a.m. Nebt-Het Hour — Journal Time for Channeling Your Inner Vision

12 – 2 p.m. Ast Hour — Journal Time for Activation

4 – 6 p.m. Het-Heru Hour — Journal Time for Inner Reflection

8 – 10 p.m. Nut Hour — Journal Time for Rest

GATEWAY 9: SACRED LOTUS INITIATION
NEFER-ATUM CONSCIOUSNESS

DAYS 64–70

Sacred Lotus Initiation Hour of Power Daily Checklist

DAY	64	65	66	67	68	69	70
4 – 6 a.m. *Nebt-Het Hour of Power* — **Journal Time for Channeling Your Inner Vision**							
Inversion (Elevate Legs on 3 Pillows)							
Hydrotherapy (Shower/Bath, Brush Teeth, Enema)							
Spiritual Observances 1–14 in the *Sacred Woman* Text for This Gateway							
Womb Yoga Fitness							
Liquid Breakfast (Freshly Pressed Fruit Juice)							
Solid Breakfast							
Herbal Tonic (Womb Care Love Herbal Detox Formula)							
Drink Water Intake: 16 oz.							

12 – 2 p.m. *Ast Hour of Power* — Journal Time for Activation

	64	65	66	67	68	69	70
Liquid Lunch (Freshly Pressed Green Juice)							
Solid Vegan Lunch							
Meditation							
Drink Water Intake: 16 oz.							

You might not complete every item every day.
These checklists serve as a guide, an invitation to complete
the practices that resonate and will help you along
your journey to healing and revitalization.

DAY	64	65	66	67	68	69	70
4 – 6 p.m. *Het-Heru Hour of Power* — Journal Time for Inner Reflection							
Liquid Dinner							
Solid Vegan Dinner							
Home Detox							
Drink Water Intake: 16 oz.							
8 – 10 p.m. *Nut Hour of Power* — Journal Time for Rest							
Healing Bath +							
Clay Application + +							
Drink Water Intake: 16 oz.							
Inversion (Elevate Legs on 3 Pillows)							
Bed Rest							

+ FOR 30 MINUTES, SOAK IN BATH WITH EPSOM OR DEAD SEA SALT.

++ APPLY WITH GAUZE; KEEP ON OVERNIGHT.

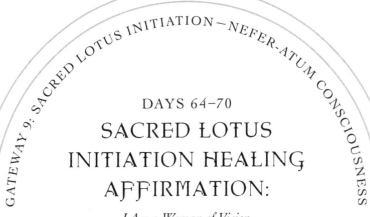

DAYS 64–70

SACRED LOTUS INITIATION HEALING AFFIRMATION:

I Am a Woman of Vision

Sacred Spirit, I thank you for showing me
the way to becoming a realized Sacred Woman.
I thank you for awakening me to my true nature,
for opening the Gateways of Sacred Woman
Enlightenment. I thank you for washing my soul at
the shore of the Great Ocean of Nu, for charging
me with the light of the sun's rays, for delivering
me a refreshed breath of life. I thank you for
helping me stand on solid ground, as I return to
my Sacred Woman seat of stability, strength, poise,
ease, and empowerment. I have gratitude, for now
I have blossomed as a Lotus of Clear Vision.

Gateway 9: Sacred Lotus Initiation

"I am a Lotus Woman emerging from the mud of overcoming.
I will blossom more beautifully each day."

DAY 64
Sacred Lotus Initiation Medicine Day

4 – 6 a.m. Nebt-Het Hour — Journal Time for Channeling Your Inner Vision

_____

_____

12 – 2 p.m. Ast Hour — Journal Time for Activation

_____

_____

4 – 6 p.m. Het-Heru Hour — Journal Time for Inner Reflection

_____

_____

8 – 10 p.m. Nut Hour — Journal Time for Rest

_____

_____

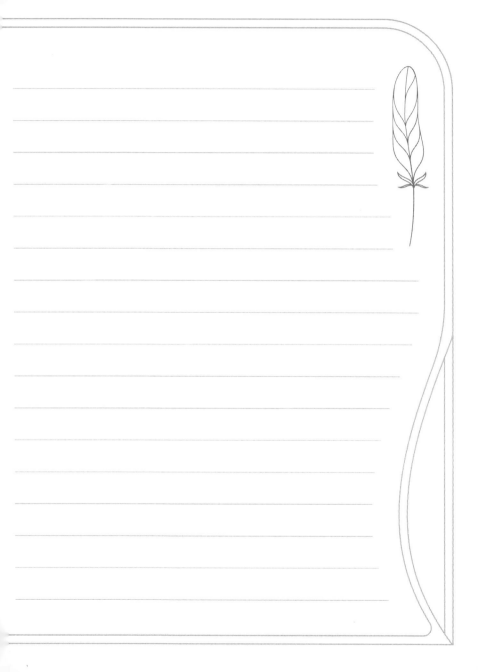

Gateway 9: Sacred Lotus Initiation

*"I am a Lotus Woman emerging from the mud of overcoming.
I will blossom more beautifully each day."*

DAY 65
Sacred Lotus Initiation Medicine Day

4 – 6 a.m. Nebt-Het Hour — Journal Time for Channeling Your Inner Vision

_____

_____

12 – 2 p.m. Ast Hour — Journal Time for Activation

_____

_____

4 – 6 p.m. Het-Heru Hour — Journal Time for Inner Reflection

_____

_____

8 – 10 p.m. Nut Hour — Journal Time for Rest

_____

_____

Gateway 9: Sacred Lotus Initiation

"I am a Lotus Woman emerging from the mud of overcoming.
I will blossom more beautifully each day."

DAY 66
Sacred Lotus Initiation Medicine Day

4 – 6 a.m. Nebt-Het Hour — Journal Time for Channeling Your Inner Vision

---

---

12 – 2 p.m. Ast Hour — Journal Time for Activation

---

4 – 6 p.m. Het-Heru Hour — Journal Time for Inner Reflection

---

8 – 10 p.m. Nut Hour — Journal Time for Rest

Gateway 9: Sacred Lotus Initiation

"I am a Lotus Woman emerging from the mud of overcoming.
I will blossom more beautifully each day."

DAY 67
Sacred Lotus Initiation Medicine Day

4 – 6 a.m. Nebt-Het Hour — Journal Time for Channeling Your Inner Vision

12 – 2 p.m. Ast Hour — Journal Time for Activation

4 – 6 p.m. Het-Heru Hour — Journal Time for Inner Reflection

8 – 10 p.m. Nut Hour — Journal Time for Rest

Gateway 9: Sacred Lotus Initiation

"I am a Lotus Woman emerging from the mud of overcoming.
I will blossom more beautifully each day."

DAY 68
Sacred Lotus Initiation Medicine Day

4 – 6 a.m. Nebt-Het Hour — Journal Time for Channeling Your Inner Vision

_____

_____

12 – 2 p.m. Ast Hour — Journal Time for Activation

_____

_____

4 – 6 p.m. Het-Heru Hour — Journal Time for Inner Reflection

_____

_____

8 – 10 p.m. Nut Hour — Journal Time for Rest

_____

_____

Gateway 9: Sacred Lotus Initiation

"I am a Lotus Woman emerging from the mud of overcoming.
I will blossom more beautifully each day."

DAY 69
Sacred Lotus Initiation Medicine Day

4 – 6 a.m. Nebt-Het Hour — Journal Time for Channeling Your Inner Vision

_____

_____

12 – 2 p.m. Ast Hour — Journal Time for Activation

_____

_____

4 – 6 p.m. Het-Heru Hour — Journal Time for Inner Reflection

_____

_____

8 – 10 p.m. Nut Hour — Journal Time for Rest

_____

_____

Gateway 9: Sacred Lotus Initiation

*"I am a Lotus Woman emerging from the mud of overcoming.
I will blossom more beautifully each day."*

DAY 70
Sacred Lotus Initiation Medicine Day

4 – 6 a.m. Nebt-Het Hour — Journal Time for Channeling Your Inner Vision

12 – 2 p.m. Ast Hour — Journal Time for Activation

4 – 6 p.m. Het-Heru Hour — Journal Time for Inner Reflection

8 – 10 p.m. Nut Hour — Journal Time for Rest

SESHAT CONSCIOUSNESS

DAYS 71–77

Sacred Time Hour of Power Daily Checklist

DAY	71	72	73	74	75	76	77
4 – 6 a.m. *Nebt-Het Hour of Power* — **Journal Time for Channeling Your Inner Vision**							
Inversion (Elevate Legs on 3 Pillows)							
Hydrotherapy (Shower/Bath, Brush Teeth, Enema)							
Spiritual Observances 1–14 in the *Sacred Woman* Text for This Gateway							
Womb Yoga Fitness							
Liquid Breakfast (Freshly Pressed Fruit Juice)							
Solid Breakfast							
Herbal Tonic (Womb Care Love Herbal Detox Formula)							
Drink Water Intake: 16 oz.							

12 – 2 p.m. *Ast Hour of Power* — **Journal Time for Activation**

	71	72	73	74	75	76	77
Liquid Lunch (Freshly Pressed Green Juice)							
Solid Vegan Lunch							
Meditation							
Drink Water Intake: 16 oz.							

You might not complete every item every day.
These checklists serve as a guide, an invitation to complete
the practices that resonate and will help you along
your journey to healing and revitalization.

DAY	71	72	73	74	75	76	77

4 – 6 p.m. *Het-Heru Hour of Power* — Journal Time for Inner Reflection

	71	72	73	74	75	76	77
Liquid Dinner							
Solid Vegan Dinner							
Home Detox							
Drink Water Intake: 16 oz.							

8 – 10 p.m. *Nut Hour of Power* — Journal Time for Rest

	71	72	73	74	75	76	77
Healing Bath +							
Clay Application ++							
Drink Water Intake: 16 oz.							
Inversion (Elevate Legs on 3 Pillows)							
Bed Rest							

+ FOR 30 MINUTES, SOAK IN BATH WITH EPSOM OR DEAD SEA SALT.
++ APPLY WITH GAUZE; KEEP ON OVERNIGHT.

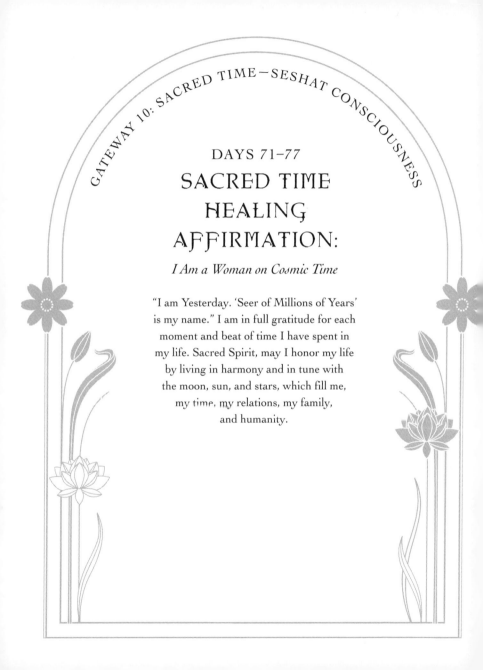

DAYS 71–77

SACRED TIME HEALING AFFIRMATION:

I Am a Woman on Cosmic Time

"I am Yesterday. 'Seer of Millions of Years'
is my name." I am in full gratitude for each
moment and beat of time I have spent in
my life. Sacred Spirit, may I honor my life
by living in harmony and in tune with
the moon, sun, and stars, which fill me,
my time, my relations, my family,
and humanity.

Gateway 10: Sacred Time

"I am that I am in harmony with Cosmic Time."

DAY 71
Sacred Time Medicine Day

4 – 6 a.m. Nebt-Het Hour — Journal Time for Channeling Your Inner Vision

_____

_____

12 – 2 p.m. Ast Hour — Journal Time for Activation

_____

_____

4 – 6 p.m. Het-Heru Hour — Journal Time for Inner Reflection

_____

_____

8 – 10 p.m. Nut Hour — Journal Time for Rest

_____

_____

Gateway 10: Sacred Time

"I am that I am in harmony with Cosmic Time."

DAY 72
Sacred Time Medicine Day

4 – 6 a.m. Nebt-Het Hour — Journal Time for Channeling Your Inner Vision

12 – 2 p.m. Ast Hour — Journal Time for Activation

4 – 6 p.m. Het-Heru Hour — Journal Time for Inner Reflection

8 – 10 p.m. Nut Hour — Journal Time for Rest

Gateway 10: Sacred Time

"I am that I am in harmony with Cosmic Time."

DAY 73
Sacred Time Medicine Day

4 – 6 a.m. Nebt-Het Hour — Journal Time for Channeling Your Inner Vision

_____

_____

12 – 2 p.m. Ast Hour — Journal Time for Activation

_____

_____

4 – 6 p.m. Het-Heru Hour — Journal Time for Inner Reflection

_____

_____

8 – 10 p.m. Nut Hour — Journal Time for Rest

_____

_____

Gateway 10: Sacred Time

"I am that I am in harmony with Cosmic Time."

DAY 74
Sacred Time Medicine Day

4 – 6 a.m. Nebt-Het Hour — Journal Time for Channeling Your Inner Vision

_____

_____

12 – 2 p.m. Ast Hour — Journal Time for Activation

_____

_____

4 – 6 p.m. Het-Heru Hour — Journal Time for Inner Reflection

_____

_____

8 – 10 p.m. Nut Hour — Journal Time for Rest

_____

_____

Gateway 10: Sacred Time

"I am that I am in harmony with Cosmic Time."

DAY 75
Sacred Time Medicine Day

4 – 6 a.m. Nebt-Het Hour — Journal Time for Channeling Your Inner Vision

12 – 2 p.m. Ast Hour — Journal Time for Activation

4 – 6 p.m. Het-Heru Hour — Journal Time for Inner Reflection

8 – 10 p.m. Nut Hour — Journal Time for Rest

Gateway 10: Sacred Time

"I am that I am in harmony with Cosmic Time."

DAY 76
Sacred Time Medicine Day

4 – 6 a.m. Nebt-Het Hour — Journal Time for Channeling Your Inner Vision

_____

_____

12 – 2 p.m. Ast Hour — Journal Time for Activation

_____

_____

4 – 6 p.m. Het-Heru Hour — Journal Time for Inner Reflection

_____

_____

8 – 10 p.m. Nut Hour — Journal Time for Rest

_____

_____

Gateway 10: Sacred Time

"I am that I am in harmony with Cosmic Time."

DAY *77*
Sacred Time Medicine Day

4 – 6 a.m. Nebt-Het Hour — Journal Time for Channeling Your Inner Vision

12 – 2 p.m. Ast Hour — Journal Time for Activation

4 – 6 p.m. Het-Heru Hour — Journal Time for Inner Reflection

8 – 10 p.m. Nut Hour — Journal Time for Rest

MESKHENET CONSCIOUSNESS

DAYS 78–84

Sacred Purpose Hour of Power Daily Checklist

DAY	78	79	80	81	82	83	84
4 – 6 a.m. *Nebt-Het Hour of Power* — **Journal Time for Channeling Your Inner Vision**							
Inversion (Elevate Legs on 3 Pillows)							
Hydrotherapy (Shower/Bath, Brush Teeth, Enema)							
Spiritual Observances 1–14 in the *Sacred Woman* Text for This Gateway							
Womb Yoga Fitness							
Liquid Breakfast (Freshly Pressed Fruit Juice)							
Solid Breakfast							
Herbal Tonic (Womb Care Love Herbal Detox Formula)							
Drink Water Intake: 16 oz.							
12 – 2 p.m. *Ast Hour of Power* — **Journal Time for Activation**							
Liquid Lunch (Freshly Pressed Green Juice)							
Solid Vegan Lunch							
Meditation							
Drink Water Intake: 16 oz.							

You might not complete every item every day.
These checklists serve as a guide, an invitation to complete
the practices that resonate and will help you along
your journey to healing and revitalization.

DAY	78	79	80	81	82	83	84

4 – 6 p.m. *Het-Heru Hour of Power* — Journal Time for Inner Reflection

	78	79	80	81	82	83	84
Liquid Dinner							
Solid Vegan Dinner							
Home Detox							
Drink Water Intake: 16 oz.							

8 – 10 p.m. *Nut Hour of Power* — Journal Time for Rest

	78	79	80	81	82	83	84
Healing Bath +							
Clay Application ++							
Drink Water Intake: 16 oz.							
Inversion (Elevate Legs on 3 Pillows)							
Bed Rest							

+ FOR 30 MINUTES, SOAK IN BATH WITH EPSOM OR DEAD SEA SALT.

++ APPLY WITH GAUZE; KEEP ON OVERNIGHT.

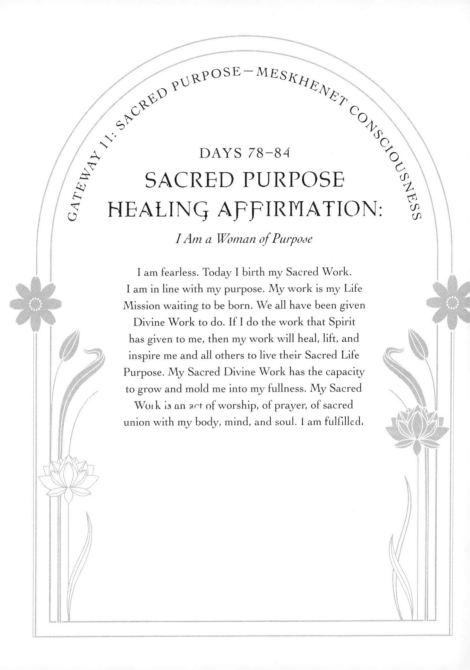

DAYS 78–84

SACRED PURPOSE

HEALING AFFIRMATION:

I Am a Woman of Purpose

I am fearless. Today I birth my Sacred Work.
I am in line with my purpose. My work is my Life
Mission waiting to be born. We all have been given
Divine Work to do. If I do the work that Spirit
has given to me, then my work will heal, lift, and
inspire me and all others to live their Sacred Life
Purpose. My Sacred Divine Work has the capacity
to grow and mold me into my fullness. My Sacred
Work is an act of worship, of prayer, of sacred
union with my body, mind, and soul. I am fulfilled.

Gateway 11: Sacred Purpose

"I am that I am living more each day my Divine Right Purpose."

DAY 78

Sacred Purpose Medicine Day

4 – 6 a.m. Nebt-Het Hour — Journal Time for Channeling Your Inner Vision

12 – 2 p.m. Ast Hour — Journal Time for Activation

4 – 6 p.m. Het-Heru Hour — Journal Time for Inner Reflection

8 – 10 p.m. Nut Hour — Journal Time for Rest

Gateway 11: Sacred Purpose

"I am that I am living more each day my Divine Right Purpose."

DAY 79
Sacred Purpose Medicine Day

4 – 6 a.m. Nebt-Het Hour — Journal Time for Channeling Your Inner Vision

_____

_____

12 – 2 p.m. Ast Hour — Journal Time for Activation

_____

_____

4 – 6 p.m. Het-Heru Hour — Journal Time for Inner Reflection

_____

_____

8 – 10 p.m. Nut Hour — Journal Time for Rest

_____

_____

Gateway 11: Sacred Purpose

"I am that I am living more each day my Divine Right Purpose."

DAY 80
Sacred Purpose Medicine Day

4 – 6 a.m. Nebt-Het Hour—Journal Time for Channeling Your Inner Vision

---

---

12 – 2 p.m. Ast Hour—Journal Time for Activation

---

4 – 6 p.m. Het-Heru Hour—Journal Time for Inner Reflection

---

8 – 10 p.m. Nut Hour—Journal Time for Rest

Gateway 11: Sacred Purpose

"I am that I am living more each day my Divine Right Purpose."

DAY 81
Sacred Purpose Medicine Day

4 – 6 a.m. Nebt-Het Hour — Journal Time for Channeling Your Inner Vision

---

12 – 2 p.m. Ast Hour — Journal Time for Activation

---

4 – 6 p.m. Het-Heru Hour — Journal Time for Inner Reflection

---

8 – 10 p.m. Nut Hour — Journal Time for Rest

Gateway 11: Sacred Purpose

"I am that I am living more each day my Divine Right Purpose."

DAY 82
Sacred Purpose Medicine Day

4 – 6 a.m. Nebt-Het Hour — Journal Time for Channeling Your Inner Vision

_____

_____

12 – 2 p.m. Ast Hour — Journal Time for Activation

_____

_____

4 – 6 p.m. Het-Heru Hour — Journal Time for Inner Reflection

_____

_____

8 – 10 p.m. Nut Hour — Journal Time for Rest

_____

_____

Gateway 11: Sacred Purpose

"I am that I am living more each day my Divine Right Purpose."

DAY 83

Sacred Purpose Medicine Day

4 – 6 a.m. Nebt-Het Hour — Journal Time for Channeling Your Inner Vision

_____

_____

12 – 2 p.m. Ast Hour — Journal Time for Activation

_____

_____

4 – 6 p.m. Het-Heru Hour — Journal Time for Inner Reflection

_____

_____

8 – 10 p.m. Nut Hour — Journal Time for Rest

_____

_____

Gateway 11: Sacred Purpose

"I am that I am living more each day my Divine Right Purpose."

DAY 84
Sacred Purpose Medicine Day

4 – 6 a.m. Nebt-Het Hour — Journal Time for Channeling Your Inner Vision

_____

_____

12 – 2 p.m. Ast Hour — Journal Time for Activation

_____

_____

4 – 6 p.m. Het-Heru Hour — Journal Time for Inner Reflection

_____

_____

8 – 10 p.m. Nut Hour — Journal Time for Rest

_____

_____

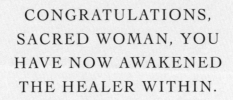

CONGRATULATIONS, SACRED WOMAN, YOU HAVE NOW AWAKENED THE HEALER WITHIN.

To the One Most High, our NTRU, our Ancestors, our Elders, and our mentors, *tua* (thank you) for walking with us, your daughters. *Mer* (love) for pouring blessings upon our journey through the pages of this journal.

Whether through your religious affiliation, spiritual direction, or cultural connections, may you be reborn and renewed. Allow your Sacred Lotus Initiation to work through you, so that you will ultimately come into the greatness of who you were destined to be. In the words of our great and beloved Ancestors, until we meet again, *hetepu*, Nefer Atum Lotus Flower Blossom.

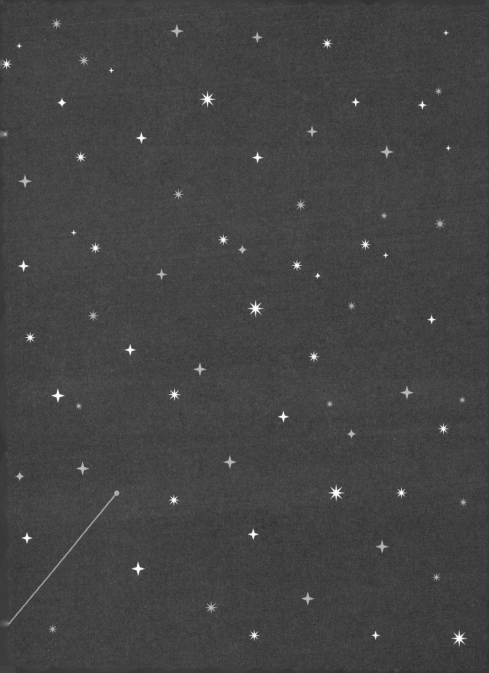

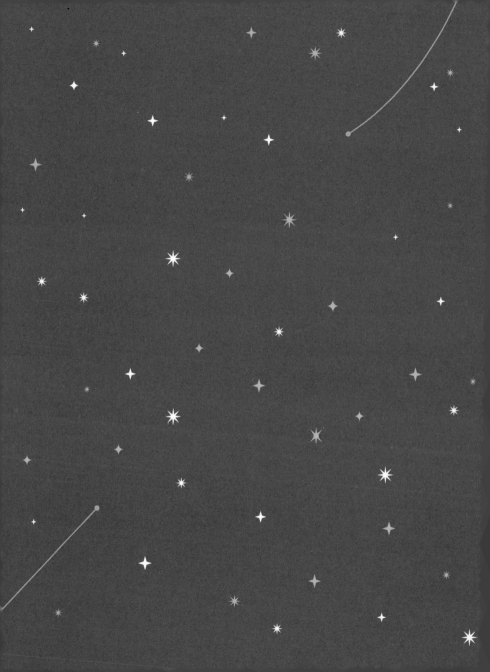